BUCKET LIST

This journal belongs to:

BUCKET LIST

If fear wasn't a factor, what would you do?

BY VIVIAN TENORIO

JAV PUBLISHING

Printed in the United Stated of America

www.viviantenorio.com

ISBN-10: 0615580734
ISBN-13: 978-0615580739

Courage is resistance to fear, mastery of fear, not absence of fear.
~Mark Twain

OTHER BOOKS BY VIVIAN TENORIO

Pink Slip to Product Launch in a Weak Economy

Pregnancy Journal: heartwarming memories

High School Journal: 4-year journal of my high school years

Dating Journal: remember why you fell in love

2012 - 2016 Gratitude Journal: magical moments should be remembered forever

2012 - 2016 Dream Journal: remember your dreams forever

My Law of Attraction Journal

My First Gratitude Journal: A write-in, draw-in gratitude journal for kids

Teen Diary

EN ESPAÑOL

Diario de Embarazo: recuerdos tiernos

2012 – 2016 Diario de Gratitud: momentos mágicos deben ser recordados para siempre

2012 – 2016 Diario de Sueños: recuerde sus suenos para siempre

The List

☐ 1. ____

☐ 2. ____

☐ 3. ____

☐ 4. ____

☐ 5. ____

☐ 6. ____

☐ 7. ____

☐ 8. ____

☐ 9. ____

☐ 10. ____

☐ 11. ____

☐ 12. ____

☐ 13. ____

☐ 14. ____

☐ 15. ____

The List

☐ 16.____

☐ 17.____

☐ 18.____

☐ 19.____

☐ 20.____

☐ 21.____

☐ 22.____

☐ 23.____

☐ 24.____

☐ 25.____

☐ 26.____

☐ 27.____

☐ 28.____

☐ 29.____

☐ 30.____

The List

- ☐ 31.______________________________________
- ☐ 32.______________________________________
- ☐ 33.______________________________________
- ☐ 34.______________________________________
- ☐ 35.______________________________________
- ☐ 36.______________________________________
- ☐ 37.______________________________________
- ☐ 38.______________________________________
- ☐ 39.______________________________________
- ☐ 40.______________________________________
- ☐ 41.______________________________________
- ☐ 42.______________________________________
- ☐ 43.______________________________________
- ☐ 44.______________________________________
- ☐ 45.______________________________________

The List

☐46.____

☐47.____

☐48.____

☐49.____

☐50.____

☐51.____

☐52.____

☐53.____

☐54.____

☐55.____

☐56.____

☐57.____

☐58.____

☐59.____

☐60.____

The List

☐61.____

☐62.____

☐63.____

☐64.____

☐65.____

☐66.____

☐67.____

☐68.____

☐69.____

☐70.____

☐71.____

☐72.____

☐73.____

☐74.____

☐75.____

The List

☐76.______________________________________

☐77.______________________________________

☐78.______________________________________

☐79.______________________________________

☐80.______________________________________

☐81.______________________________________

☐82.______________________________________

☐83.______________________________________

☐84.______________________________________

☐85.______________________________________

☐86.______________________________________

☐87.______________________________________

☐88.______________________________________

☐89.______________________________________

☐90.______________________________________

The List

☐91.____

☐92.____

☐93.____

☐94.____

☐95.____

☐96.____

☐97.____

☐98.____

☐99.____

☐100.____

☐ 1 *Date Completed* / /

☐ 2 *Date Completed* / /

☐ 3 *Date Completed* / /

☐ 4 *Date Completed* / /

☐ 5 *Date Completed* / /

☐ 6 *Date Completed* / /

☐ 7 *Date Completed* / /

☐ 8 *Date Completed* / /

☐ 9 *Date Completed* / /

☐ 10 *Date Completed* / /

☐ 11 *Date Completed* / /

☐ 12 *Date Completed* / /

☐ 13 *Date Completed* / /

☐ 14 *Date Completed* / /

☐ 15 *Date Completed* / /

☐ 16 *Date Completed* / /

How are you feeling?

☐ 17 *Date Completed* / /

☐ 18 *Date Completed* / /

☐ 19 *Date Completed* / /

☐ 20 *Date Completed* / /

☐ 21 *Date Completed* / /

☐ 22 *Date Completed* / /

☐ 23 *Date Completed* / /

☐ 24 *Date Completed* / /

☐ 25 *Date Completed* / /

☐ 26 *Date Completed* / /

☐ 27 *Date Completed* / /

☐ 28 *Date Completed* / /

How are you feeling?

☐ 29 *Date Completed* / /

☐ 30 *Date Completed* / /

☐ 31 *Date Completed* / /

☐ 32 *Date Completed* / /

☐ 33 *Date Completed* / /

☐ 34 *Date Completed* / /

☐ 35 *Date Completed* / /

☐ 36 *Date Completed* / /

☐ 37 *Date Completed* / /

☐ 38 *Date Completed* / /

☐ 39 *Date Completed* / /

☐ 40 *Date Completed* / /

How are you feeling?

☐ 41 *Date Completed* / /

☐ 42 *Date Completed* / /

☐ 43 *Date Completed* / /

☐ 44 *Date Completed* / /

☐ 45 *Date Completed* / /

☐ 46 *Date Completed* / /

☐ 47 *Date Completed* / /

☐ 48 *Date Completed* / /

How are you feeling?

☐ 49 *Date Completed* / /

☐ 50 *Date Completed* / /

☐ 51 *Date Completed* / /

☐ 52 *Date Completed* / /

☐ 53 *Date Completed* / /

☐ 54 *Date Completed* / /

☐ 55 *Date Completed* / /

☐ 56 *Date Completed* / /

How are you feeling?

☐ 57 *Date Completed* / /

☐ 58 *Date Completed* / /

☐ 59 *Date Completed* / /

☐ 60 *Date Completed* / /

☐ 61 *Date Completed* / /

☐ 62 *Date Completed* / /

How are you feeling?

☐ 63 *Date Completed* / /

☐ 64 *Date Completed* / /

☐ 65 *Date Completed* / /

☐ 66 *Date Completed* / /

☐ 67 *Date Completed* / /

☐ 68 *Date Completed* / /

How are you feeling?

☐ 69 *Date Completed* / /

☐ 70 *Date Completed* / /

☐ 71 *Date Completed* / /

☐ 72 *Date Completed* / /

☐ 73 *Date Completed* / /

☐ 74 *Date Completed* / /

How are you feeling?

☐ 75 *Date Completed* / /

☐ 76 *Date Completed* / /

☐ 77 *Date Completed* / /

☐ 78 *Date Completed* / /

☐ 79 *Date Completed* / /

☐ 80 *Date Completed* / /

How are you feeling?

☐ 81 *Date Completed* / /

☐ 82 *Date Completed* / /

☐ 83 *Date Completed* / /

☐ 84 *Date Completed* / /

☐ 85 *Date Completed* / /

☐ 86 *Date Completed* / /

How are you feeling?

☐ 87 *Date Completed* / /

☐ 88 *Date Completed* / /

☐ 89 *Date Completed* / /

☐ 90 *Date Completed* / /

☐ 91 *Date Completed* / /

☐ 92 *Date Completed* / /

How are you feeling?

☐ 93 *Date Completed* / /

☐ 94 *Date Completed* / /

☐ 95 *Date Completed* / /

☐ 96 *Date Completed* / /

☐ 97 *Date Completed* / /

☐ 98 *Date Completed* / /

☐ 99 *Date Completed* / /

☐ 100 *Date Completed* / /

How do you feel now that you have completed your list?

BUCKET LIST

Was there one item on your list that you wish you have NOT completed?

BUCKET LIST

Was there one item on your list that you wish you had completed years ago?

BUCKET LIST

How has your list changed you?

BUCKET LIST

Notes

Notes

Notes

Notes

Notes

Notes

Notes

Notes

Notes

Notes

Notes

Notes

Notes

Notes

Notes

Notes

Notes

Notes

Notes

Notes

Notes

Notes

ABOUT THE AUTHOR

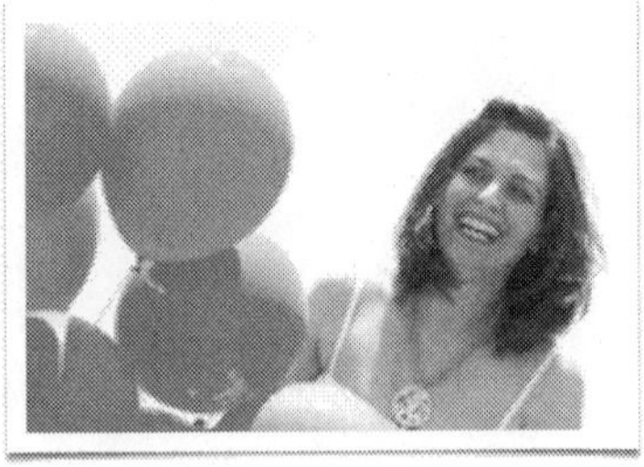

Vivian's belief in thinking that anything was possible if she just put her mind to it helped her deal with and hustle through the challenges she faced as a teenage mother, young wife and high school dropout.

This no-limits attitude led her to open a restaurant, start Signature Flan, start a publishing company "JAV Publishing", and become the author of her 1st book and now creator of a series of journals.